the pilates

difference

the pilates
difference

Jennifer Dufton

hamlyn

Jennifer Dufton is a fully qualified Pilates teacher and has a Pilates studio in North Norfolk. Before moving to Norfolk, she taught Pilates in some of London's most prestigious studios including the Chelsea Harbour Club, Triyoga in Primrose Hill, the Pilates Studio in Great Portland Street and the Westminster Physiotherapy Centre. She has worked with a wide range of clients including actors, models, musicians and members of the Royal Ballet. She is a member of The PILATESfoundation® UK, having trained with one of its co-founders, Anne-Marie Zulkahari. She also qualified with Alan Herdman Studios, and with the International Body Arts and Science Teacher Training Programme under Rael Isacowitz.

First published in Great Britain in 2003 by
Hamlyn, a division of Octopus Publishing Group Ltd
2–4 Heron Quays, London E14 4JP

© Octopus Publishing Group Ltd 2003

Jennifer Dufton has asserted her moral right to be identified as the author of this work.

ISBN 0 600 60788 7

A CIP catalogue record for this book is available from the British Library

Printed and bound in China

10   9   8   7   6   5   4   3

SAFETY NOTE

It is advisable to check with your doctor first before embarking on any exercise programme. Pilates should not be regarded as a replacement for professional medical treatment, a physician should be consulted in all matters relating to health and particularly in respect of pregnancy and any symptoms which may require diagnosis or medical attention. While the advice and information in this book is believed to be accurate and the instructions given have been devised to avoid strain, neither the author nor the publisher can accept any legal responsibility for any injury sustained while following the exercises.

Anyone who is pregnant or trying to conceive is advised not to attempt the exercises in this book. Although Pilates may be safely practised during pregnancy and also postnatally, only do so under the supervision of your doctor and a qualified Pilates teacher.

Prolonged sitting in poor posture will usually cause your abdominals to weaken, the muscles in the backs of your legs to shorten, your spine to slump, and your shoulders to round forwards. This can lead to lower backache, and chronic neck and shoulder pain. If you are spending long periods sitting badly, the chances are you need to improve your posture and your flexibility.

A well-moving joint is a well-lubricated joint. When your joint moves, it releases synovial fluid, which works like oil on a rusty hinge. When you do Pilates exercises in a slow, controlled manner, you increase synovial fluid production, whether it is in the spine, hips, shoulders or elbows. This keeps your joints flexible, protects them from seizing up and decreasing your range of movement, and may help to prevent arthritis.

Pilates aims to improve what is known as **Functional Flexibility**. This means getting as flexible as you can be, without sacrificing muscle strength and therefore good alignment in the process. To perform at its best, your body needs **optimum Functional Flexibility** and **optimum Functional Strength**. No more, and no less. This is very different from many other exercise regimes and aims to keep your body perfectly balanced.

better body alignment

In addition to sitting in poor posture, are you using the same muscles over and over again? Do you always hold a telephone with the same hand or carry your shoulderbag or briefcase on the same side? Repetitive movements affect the symmetry of your body so that you become more developed on one side than the other. Your body may fall into bad patterns of behaviour, which can affect your posture and muscle balance and lead to aches and pains. Pilates rebalances your muscles for better body alignment, and in doing so improves your posture.

postural benefits

- **Weak muscles become strong.**

- **Chronically overused muscles learn to relax.**

- **Rounded shoulders begin to open and drop down.**

- **Collapsed stomach muscles lift and strengthen to support your spine.**

- **A slumped spine lengthens and straightens.**

- **A rigid spine softens and regains its natural curves.**

less stress, more vitality

If your life seems to grow ever more stressful, you need to manage stress better if it is not to control your life. With Pilates, the combination of focusing your mind, breathing well, and relaxing and moving your body, greatly reduces the effects of stress. Many people also find their blood pressure lowers through regular Pilates practice.

View your Pilates practice as a safe haven. Use your sessions to grab some time for yourself, to unwind, de-stress and revive. When you finish, you'll feel relaxed, reinvigorated, more grounded and ready to face new challenges.

healing with pilates

Your body stores all your emotions, whether good or bad, and this affects your posture. You hold your body differently when you are happy from when you are sad or angry and if you sustain a particular emotion for a long time, your body may retain that posture. For example, if someone feels a need to be protected, they may frequently round their shoulders forwards to protect their centre. Over time, their pectoral muscles become short and tight, resulting in a permanently round-shouldered posture. Learning to be aware of your body doesn't just mean learning how it moves, but also how it feels.

Through trauma, apathy or neglect, your muscles can lose their strength, ligaments lose their elasticity and connective tissue hardens. Since Pilates calls upon the mind to move muscles with precision, it can help you to become more aware of the subtle connection between body and mind. By releasing our bodies through exercise, perhaps we can also heal our minds.

increase mental alertness

Breathing well improves the quality of your blood supply and therefore your level of alertness. By breathing well in Pilates, you will clear your mind and leave it more able to take in and process new information. In Pilates exercises you are often co-ordinating complex movement. This focus should help to keep your mental powers in good order as you grow older.

improve your self-esteem

✓ Greater sense of pride in yourself.

✓ Improved self-confidence.

Regularly taking time to do something that makes you feel good enhances the rest of your life. You feel a sense of pride in your body every time it performs a movement that you previously thought would be impossible, such as touching your toes. The fact that you achieved this by connecting your mind and body gives you an amazing sense of empowerment. In addition, you become more accepting of your imperfections. What used to bug you about your body becomes one of the areas you're still working on and in which you expect to see results with continued practice.

The better you feel about yourself, the more you want to exercise and eat healthily. Feeling good about your body, whatever your size and shape, gives a new sense of self-assurance that attracts people to you. Self-confidence also happens to be the strongest aphrodisiac there is.

acquire a feeling of wellbeing

When you really concentrate on each exercise, you begin to understand what people mean when they talk about 'being in the flow'. You suddenly find yourself living fully in the present, not worrying about the future, nor feeling regretful about the past. The more this effect spills over into your daily life, the more able you are to *stay* in the moment. This fosters an innate sense of wellbeing. You become a better listener, you are more perceptive and more aware. You are more successful at work and in your relationships – you are happier. This sense of happiness stems from the quality of your movements in Pilates. At last you are in control of your body, and you are in tune with what you are doing.

Pilates can also improve your sex life, your circulation, and give you clearer, more radiant skin. Do you need any more reasons to start your programme?

no such thing as a quick fix

Let's get real here. There is no such thing as a quick fix in any exercise regime. Pilates will give you fabulous improvements in body and mind over time, but it is not going to give you supermodel or film star looks overnight. Instead of searching for the impossible dream of perfection, aim to get the best body you possibly can. One that moves with grace and ease, one that looks strong, toned, flexible and sexy. In thirty sessions you will start to see changes, but you need to continue with Pilates to see continued improvements.

Pilates will sculpt long, lean muscles. It will also increase your lean muscle mass, which means your body burns up calories faster, helping you to lose weight and keep it off, if that's what your body needs. Many people find they go down a clothing size without changing their eating habits.

If you are overweight, and want to speed up weight loss, you should combine Pilates with a healthy diet and some cardiovascular exercise, to help reduce your body fat. Pilates can give you a cardiovascular workout at its more advanced level, but to begin with beginners will need to supplement their classes.

Cardiovascular exercise need only be moderate. You will achieve results from a 30- to 60-minute session, three to five times per week, of brisk walking, swimming or any other activity that raises the heart rate. You could do this after your Pilates routine three times per week, or exercise every day and alternate a Pilates class one day with cardio the next.

Forget crash diets, be honest with yourself – you know they don't work. As soon as you go back to your normal way of eating, the weight piles back on. Read books on healthy eating or visit a nutritionist and start to eat well. That usually means increasing fruit and vegetables in your diet, eating lean meat/fish/soya and smaller portions of complex carbohydrates. You'll also need to cut down on processed foods, saturated fats and sugars, but there's no harm in giving yourself the odd treat every once in a while, to keep you going. Do all that and the weight will almost certainly come off.

get the balance right

Quite simply, if the energy going in is less than the energy expended you'll lose weight. If it doesn't, you'll either need to eat a little less, or exercise a little more. It isn't easy, and it's certainly not the way we would choose to eat if all foods were equal, but if we want to lose weight and keep it off, sadly that's the bottom line. Whatever you decide to do, try to find a healthy way of eating that honestly suits your lifestyle and includes foods that you actually like. It may sound daft, but you'll be amazed at how many people don't take either of these factors into account and wonder why they fail. Choosing something you can stick to is the best way of ensuring success.

The best rate of weight loss is 0.5–1 kg (1–2 lbs) a week, as this means you'll lose body fat rather than lean muscle and are more likely to keep the weight off. If you lose weight at that rate while taking your thirty Pilates classes spread over 10 weeks, you could safely lose up to 10 kg (20 lbs) by your thirtieth session.

Pilates principles

In Pilates, quality of movement is emphasized over mindless repetition, and this is achieved by following six fundamental principles: breathing, concentration, control, centring, precision and flow. Remember that it takes time to improve body awareness and to lengthen and strengthen muscles, so be patient. Keep referring back to these principles and, in time, you'll feel them within your body as you move.

breathing

Breathing is essential to life, so breathing well is vital. Many of us shallow-breathe, or don't fully expel the air from our lungs, so we almost never get a good breath of fresh air. Breathing better will:

✓ Improve your circulation.

✓ Rid your body of toxins.

✓ Improve your skin tone.

✓ Encourage concentration and help you to recruit the appropriate muscles for your movements.

✓ Calm your body and mind.

✓ Help you control your movements in daily life.

concentration

This is the key to connecting mind and body. It's the mind that makes the body move. Concentrate on each part of every exercise: the rhythm of your breath, the position of your head, the curve of your back, the bend in your legs, the straightness of your arms, etc. Pay attention to the individual muscles you are working and they will fire up with extra strength. As your concentration improves, you'll gain a heightened sense of body awareness so that you can recognize body

sensation far more accurately. This new skill is essential for improving your Pilates technique and it's great for enhancing your sex life, too.

control

One of the most vital elements of Pilates is controlling your movements properly – Joseph Pilates originally called his new exercise programme 'Contrology'. It is better to perform two exercise repetitions correctly, than twenty incorrectly. Badly performed exercises are the primary cause of injuries in other exercise methods. By carefully controlling your muscles, Pilates becomes one of the safest exercise programmes around. Control is also required to ensure you get the maximum benefit from each exercise. Each detail of every movement serves a function.

centring

Think about the way you move: which muscles do you use most frequently? Most probably the muscles of your arms and legs. But there is a large group of muscles in the centre of your body – starting from the pelvic floor muscles and including the muscles in the buttocks, hips, stomach and back, all the way up to the lower ribs – which we all too often neglect. Joseph Pilates called this centre the powerhouse (see page 18), and it is your powerhouse that you need

Used to keep the spine upright. The deep multifidus in the lumbo-sacral region plays a vital role in maintaining core stability along with the abdominal muscles.

8 Quadratus lumborum (not shown) or 'lower back' muscle, a deep muscle at the side of the waist. *Used* primarily for side-bending.

9 Gluteus maximus forms the greater part of the buttock muscles. *Used* for running, jumping and climbing.

10 Hamstrings three muscles that run down the back of the thigh.

Used to lift the thigh backward away from the body, and to bend the leg at the knee.

11 Gastrocnemius forms the greater part of the calf muscles, and runs down the back of the lower leg. *Used* for flexing the foot.

12 Pectorals these chest muscles bring the arm towards the body. *Used* to rotate the arm, and flex and stabilise the shoulder.

13 Biceps muscle of the upper arm. *Used* to bend the elbow.

14 Rectus abdominis or 'six pack'

muscles, run down the front of the abdomen. *Used* to bend the trunk, pulling the lower body toward the ribcage. Help to maintain good posture, working together with the deeper transversus abdominis (not shown) and the obliques.

15 External obliques abdominal muscles running diagonally along the sides of the trunk. *Used* to bend and rotate the trunk, working with the deeper internal obliques (not shown) and the rectus abdominis. Important for core stability.

16 Psoas (not shown) or 'hip flexor'. Two deep muscles running from the front of the femur, through the pelvis, to the lumbar region of the spine. *Used* to flex the thigh. Important for good pelvic stability.

17 Adductors four inner thigh muscles. *Used* for moving the leg inward.

18 Quadriceps or 'quads'. The quadriceps femoris is one muscle with four heads and runs down the front of the thigh. *Used* to perform the opposite movement to the hamstrings, extending or straightening the knee. It also acts on the hip joint to raise the thigh towards the hip.

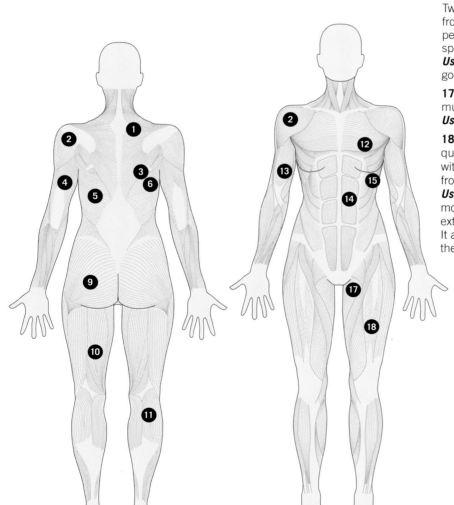

core stabilization

Core stabilization is the key to Pilates. You need to strengthen your trunk, your 'centre', in order to move most efficiently. If your centre is strong, you are better balanced and this will have a dramatic impact on the rest of the body.

In core stabilization exercises, you create a 'girdle of strength', the powerhouse, around your trunk to protect your spine and your internal organs. This can then be called upon to control your limbs while protecting your spine.

Many of us exercise without thinking about the beginning of each movement. As a result, we move poorly which puts us at risk of straining our muscles or giving ourselves an even greater injury. Pilates will train you to recruit your powerhouse at the beginning of each movement. In each exercise, you start by strengthening your centre before working any of the other muscles. In this way, you learn to initiate from the centre of your body. This powerful technique will:

✓ Improve your alignment and posture.

✓ Radically reduce back pain.

✓ Strengthen and protect your body for life.

the powerhouse muscles

Joseph Pilates originally described this region as lying between the base of the ribs and the top of the pelvis, but nowadays the powerhouse refers to the area from the lower ribcage to the pelvic floor. Your abdominal muscles surround and support your lower torso and connect your pelvis to your ribs. The most important abdominal muscles (see diagram, right) form a corset that stabilizes your spine, protects your internal organs and enables you to bend and twist.

The **rectus abdominis** is the easiest abdominal muscle to activate but it needs to be controlled by the deeper abdominal muscles, the **transversus abdominis** and the **internal** and **external obliques**. These are usually the weakest and can often be forgotten when doing stomach crunches in the gym. For this reason, in Pilates you will work from the inside out, starting with the deeper layers of muscle and moving outward towards the more superficial muscle. You can only activate the deeper muscles by breathing well and that's why breathing plays such an important part in Pilates. Strengthening all your abdominal muscles, and not just the rectus abdominis, will make all the difference to achieving that firmer, flatter stomach.

Other muscles also play a key role in core stabilization. These include the muscles of your back, buttocks, your hip flexors and even your pelvic floor. They work in conjuction with the abdominal muscles to stabilize your core. Pilates will strengthen every one of them and teach you to use them correctly when you move.

the abdominal muscles

transversus abdominis ▶

◀ internal obliques

◀ external obliques

◀ rectus abdominis

inner

outer

shoulder stabilization

It is very common to overuse your deep supporting shoulder muscles or use them incorrectly, and this frequently leads to stiff, painful shoulders, plus chronic neck pain and headaches. Good shoulder stabilization will help to reduce these problems.

how to stabilize your shoulders

Holding your shoulder blades stable when you move allows your arms to reach or lift freely. Throughout this book, you'll be instructed to stabilize your shoulders, or slide your shoulder blades down into your back. To do this, think of drawing down the outsides of your shoulder blades so that they move downwards towards your hips, or imagine you are sliding your armpits down towards your hips. Don't let the shoulder blades retract together as you perform the movement. They mustn't protrude or 'wing'. Instead, as you slide them down, think of them wrapping forwards slightly towards the side of the ribcage. It's a small but vital movement.

As you exercise, if a movement is tricky to perform, you may find your shoulders are the first area to tense up. Rather than allowing this to happen, you need consciously to relax your shoulders during all the movements, by sliding the shoulder blade down your back.

1 Stand in front of a mirror and slowly extend one arm forwards and up to the ceiling. Now slowly take that straight arm down.

2 Examine that movement. When you lifted the arm above your head, was there space between the top of the shoulder and your ear? (See above left.) Or did your shoulder move up towards your ear creating tension? (See above right.)

3 Try raising your arm again and this time focus on sliding the outside edge of the shoulder blade gently down and then lift your arm. This gives more space between the top of the shoulder and the ear and creates no tension. If you can only move your shoulder and arm up together, the joint is not working as it should. Pilates should help to free it up.

pelvic floor

The pelvic floor muscles are a sling of muscles in the pelvic area that support the internal organs and connect to the rest of the abdominal region. They are extremely important as they are fundamental to core stability and also interact with the thoracic region (the part of the body enclosed by the ribs), affecting your ability to breathe.

The pelvic floor is just like any other muscle. If you don't exercise it, it grows weak and can lead to problems. If your pelvic floor loses tone and elasticity, your posture collapses, your stomach protrudes, and the muscles that control your rectum, bladder, and your vagina, if you are a woman, weaken. A weak pelvic floor can lead to back pain and also incontinence (most often experienced by women after childbirth).

Since the outer muscles of the pelvic floor surround the sexual organs, strong pelvic floor muscles can also help sustain your libido. Improve your pelvic floor muscles, and you could also improve your sex life!

It helps to incorporate the pelvic floor in lateral breathing (see page 23).

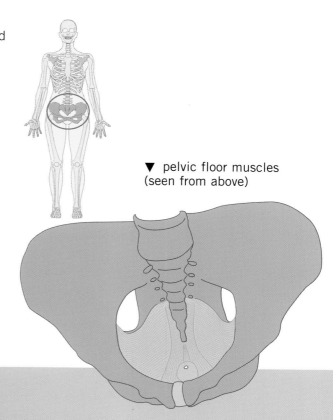

▼ pelvic floor muscles
(seen from above)

how to find your pelvic floor

The easiest way for both men and women to find their pelvic floor is to stop the flow of urine briefly while urinating. The pelvic floor is the muscle you'll feel when you stop the flow. Try this a couple of times, just so you can locate it, but not on a regular basis as frequently stopping urine flow may not be good for your bladder in the long term.

• Learn to engage your pelvic floor muscles when you are standing, sitting or lying down.

• Practise gently engaging and releasing your pelvic floor muscles regularly so that you can locate them easily. Women usually find it easiest to locate them if they imagine sucking water up into their vaginas.

Men are lifting their urethas and need only remember the feeling they get when they walk into icy cold seawater. Recreating that 'lift' works the pelvic floor muscle. Remember not to engage your buttock muscles as you lift.

breathing

If we breathe poorly, our lungs don't take in enough fresh oxygen for optimum health,

the ribcage region can become stiff and inflexible and this can lead to back problems.

If we breathe well, we oxygenate the blood, dispel toxins and our circulation improves.

There are different ways of breathing badly. Some people are upper-chest breathers and take short shallow breaths, tightening the neck and the throat, lifting the shoulders and ribs with each inhalation. This is particularly stressful on the body and is very common among asthma sufferers. Others tend to be more diaphragmatic breathers, only filling out their stomachs with each breath.

lateral breathing

In Pilates, we practise what is known as lateral breathing as this provides greater **core stability**. By breathing more laterally, we expand our ribcage sideways with each breath, breathing air into the sides and back of the ribcage. This works the muscles between the ribs, facilitating their expansion, making the upper body more flexible.

1 Place your hands on either side of your ribcage. **Breathe in slowly and gently** through your nose, allowing your ribs to expand outwards laterally into your hands, as you try to fill the sides and back of your ribcage with air. Don't force the movement, your ribcage may only move slightly at first.

2 **Exhale slowly** through the mouth keeping your lips and jaw relaxed so that the lips are not pursed together and the jaw is not clenched.

3 Take 6–10 breaths in this manner.

4 Repeat 6–10 breaths but this time just allow your arms to rest by your sides.

It can take a while for lateral breathing to come naturally, particularly if your upper and mid-back are tight. Just keep practising and it will eventually become second nature.

important note

The style of breathing described in this book is the basic way of Pilates breathing. It has been kept deliberately simple since you are learning at home without the benefit of supervised instruction. If you feel you have fallen into bad breathing habits and can't seem to get the hang of lateral breathing even after practising diligently, it would be well worth taking a private lesson with a Pilates instructor who would be able to teach you better breathing.

drawing in the abdominals

When we breathe laterally in Pilates, we also incorporate the abdominal muscles and pelvic floor in our movements for even greater core stability.

Breathing this way will feel very different to start with, but keep practising the method described below. To begin with, you may find you inhale into your upper chest or your stomach as well as into your ribcage. That's fine for now – if your ribcage is stiff and inflexible, it may take a while before it begins to move more freely. Try lateral breathing and drawing in the abdominals while sitting and standing, as well as lying down. This will strengthen your deep abdominal muscles, which have probably been underused. These are the muscles that will help to give you a flat stomach and protect you from lower back pain.

If you are finding it difficult to locate your pelvic floor muscles, or can't seem to be able to engage them smoothly and gently without tightening your buttock muscles, then just leave the pelvic floor out for the moment and focus on drawing in the abdominals correctly on each exhalation. You can always go back to incorporating the pelvic floor when you become more experienced.

1 Lie on your back, with your knees bent at a 90-degree angle, and your feet and knees hip-width apart. Rest your arms by your sides. **Inhale** gently through the nose, taking the breath in laterally, filling the sides and back of your ribcage with air. Pause momentarily.

2 As you start to **exhale slowly** through the mouth, gently engage your pelvic floor, and as you **exhale**, feel your lower stomach start to sink down towards the floor. As you **continue to exhale**, allow your stomach to sink down a little further by drawing in your lower stomach muscles. Your stomach will hollow out. Don't brace your stomach muscles, just sink them gently downwards and make sure you don't move your spine. Pause momentarily.

3 Gently **inhale** through your nose into the sides and back of your ribcage. Pause momentarily, then repeat the exhalation as above.

Repeat for 6–10 full breaths.

neutral spine

Most of the exercises in this book are performed in what is known as 'neutral spine'

position. This describes the natural curves of your back and is usually the best position

for your spine, as it places the least stress on the spine and therefore protects the back.

finding your neutral spine

Neutral spine allows the best alignment of the body so that the muscles are well balanced. It also ensures you are engaging your abdominal muscles correctly. It is unique to the individual, so finding the position that is right for you may take a little practice.

✗ Lie down on the floor with your knees bent. If you tilt your pelvis up (by rocking your pubic bone up towards the ceiling), you will lose the natural curve in your back as your spine flattens into the floor and your tailbone lifts off it.

✗ If you tilt your pelvis the other way (by rocking your pubic bone down to the floor), your back overarches.

✓ The neutral spine position lies between these two positions. Your pelvis is balanced so that the curve in your lower spine behind your waist is not completely lost by pressing your back into the floor, nor is your back overarched leaving a big gap between your back and the floor.

When you are in neutral, your tailbone (coccyx) remains on the floor and lengthens away, and your pubic bone and two hipbones are level with each other. Everyone's position will be slightly different, but in most cases there should be just

enough room for someone to slide a flat hand in the slight gap behind your waist when you are in neutral spine.

In Pilates, you want to work in neutral spine when you are standing, sitting or lying down with your feet on the floor. If your feet are lifted off the mat, then you can come out of neutral and allow your lower back to press into the floor for additional support.

spinal articulation

Your spine is made up of 24 small bones (vertebrae) plus your sacrum and coccyx

bones. The bones of the spine support your torso and protect your spinal cord.

They also allow you to move. A flexible spine lets you twist, turn and spiral in many

different directions.

To create a flexible spine, you need to stretch and articulate it. You also need to strengthen it to improve your posture. Many Pilates exercises work on strengthening and increasing flexibility in the spine. In many of them you will read expressions such as 'roll down the spine', 'curl up the spine', or 'peel the spine off the mat one vertebra at a time'. All this really means is articulating your spine so that you work through each section of the spine, mobilizing and separating each vertebra so they move one at a time.

As you curl up and down your spine, you will be aware that some sections feel flexible, while others feel stiff and tight, and hard to separate from each other. These tight areas are the areas you must really focus on, taking your time, and breathing slowly to increase the opening of the area. Whether you are rolling up or down, imagine you are curving your spine into the shape of a letter C each time you move, as this will help you to articulate better through the spine thus increasing flexibility and strength.

alignment

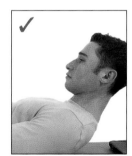

head position

Crunching the vertebra at the back of your neck can lead to neck and shoulder tension, pain and poor posture. When **sitting** or **standing**, think of lengthening through the crown of your head to elongate the back of your neck. *Imagine a piece of rope attached to your crown being gently drawn up to the ceiling.*

When **lying** on your back, use a head rest for support and gently elongate the back of your neck. Lower your chin slightly towards your chest, but still leave a gap the size of a peach between your chin and chest.

If your head and shoulders are **lifted** off the mat, lengthen through the crown of the head to elongate the back of your neck. Your head should be above your breastbone with a peach-sized gap between chin and chest. Your abdominal muscles and the back of your chest support you so you don't strain the neck muscles.

ribcage

Sticking the ribs out and up when raising the arms will cause you to arch your lower back and strain your neck and shoulders. If you notice your ribs 'popping out', correct this by gently sliding your ribcage down the front of your body towards your hips. This lengthens your spine and stops your back arching.

turning the legs out

Occasionally, you'll be asked to turn your legs out. This position involves rotating your thighs outwards in the hip sockets so that your heels come together, and very gently engaging the lower part of your buttocks as if you were holding a coin between them. If you do this correctly, you will also feel the muscles at the top of your inner thighs engage. If you are lying down, try not to lift your tailbone as you engage but lengthen your legs away from you to keep your leg muscles stretched. Working in this turned out position ensures that you work the correct muscles to tone up your hips, buttocks and thighs and stabilize your lower body.

working in opposition

Muscles tend to work in pairs or groups. For example, if you lift one arm up and bend it at the elbow, your bicep muscle at the front of your upper arm is working to make the bending movement. For the movement to happen, however, the muscle at the back of your upper arm (the tricep) has to lengthen to allow the bicep to bend.

Other muscles in your body also have to work when you bend your arm to stop your whole body bending over with it. These are called stabilizer muscles. If one muscle reaches away from your body, at least one other also has to work to keep your body counter-balanced so that you don't tip over. As you practice Pilates, you will need to train yourself to emphasize these opposing movements.

body alignment

When you are performing the exercises, it is essential that you do them symmetrically so that your body develops symmetrically. Imagine a square in the centre of your body that runs from shoulder to shoulder, shoulder to hip, hip to hip, and shoulder to hip. Try to keep this square shape, or 'box' as it is sometimes called, as you perform the exercises.

People often favour one side of the body more than the other and being aware of this will keep you in alignment, so that you don't lean over too far to one side, or twist too far to the other as you exercise.

preparation week

Don't be in a hurry to advance into your Pilates programme. The best way to begin is to lay the foundations first. Read the Introduction a few times and practise the basics (see opposite). Don't worry if it doesn't all make complete sense immediately. As you begin to practise Pilates, it will all start to fall into place.

Ideally, one week before you start your Pilates programme, try lateral breathing (see page 22) and drawing in the abdominal muscles (see page 23). Try 10 full breath cycles (breathing in and out is one full cycle) three times per day. Breathing like this for a week before you begin your programme will begin to strengthen those deep abdominal muscles that are so important for your posture. If you can begin to do this before you start, you'll find you progress far more quickly.

what you need
the space

Choose a warm, quiet space where you like to be and that you can make your own three times a week. If you can keep your mat out all the time, so that you're already set up, so much the better. You may wish to add candles and flowers, and play some quiet relaxing music. Make the space as much of a sanctuary as you can, so that you'll want to come in and practise. If you can only find space by clearing away the kids' toys in front of the sofa, that's fine. Make the area as comfortable as it can be, and then just start.

the mat

Use a mat to protect your spine. A Pilates mat is ideal, but you can use a yoga mat, which is slightly thinner. You can purchase either at most sports shops. If a mat is not available, use blankets or towels to create a cushioned surface on which you can lie full-length. A surface that is too soft is not good as it may inhibit balance and make it hard to control your movements.

the head rest

For all the exercises performed lying down, it is useful to use a head rest. This will support the head, and help to lengthen the neck, relax the shoulders and facilitate better breathing. Either use a book, about an inch thick and large enough to place your head on without it rolling off, or make your own head rest by using an inch-thick cut of foam. When you are more experienced, you may no longer need a head rest, but it is very helpful for your first 30 Pilates sessions.

frequency

Practise your routine three times per week, ideally leaving one day in between for the body to rest. Try to stick to a regular Monday/Wednesday/Friday or a regular Tuesday/Thursday/Sunday pattern, if you can. The more you can make it a routine, the more easily Pilates will become a habit for life. If you have to miss a day, just make sure you make up for it later in the week so, even if you end up having to practise two days in a row, you still complete your three sessions that week.

maintaining motivation

If it's your regular day to practise and you don't feel like it, try striking a deal with yourself: you just have to lie down on the mat and do one exercise. If, after that, you still don't feel like exercising, that's fine, you can leave it for that day. The chances are, the first exercise will start to feel so good that, before you know it, you'll want to continue.

basics to practise before you start

● **Find neutral spine (see page 24).**

● **Find your pelvic floor (see page 21).**

● **Practise lateral breathing (see page 22).**

● **Practise drawing in your abdominals (see page 23).**

● **Check out your shoulder stabilization (see page 20).**

● **Practise your standing posture (see page 15).**

● **Learn how to lengthen the back of your neck (see pages 26).**

following the programme

A full programme of exercises takes you through your first thirty Pilates lessons and beyond. Everyone should start at Level 1 and work through all three levels, doing the exercises in the given order. Exercises range from beginners' to early intermediate and can be tailored to suit individual needs.

doing the exercises

Everyone's body is different and you will find some exercises challenge your own particular body structure more than others. That's fine. There is no competition and no rush. Go at your own pace, only progressing according to the instructions given when you are sure your body is ready to move on. When you first perform an exercise, stick to the low end of the range of repetitions given. Only when you are sure you have mastered it should you do the top number of recommended repetitions. Never do more than suggested. It's like doubling your medication to get better quicker, it won't give you better results!

transitions

At the end of each exercise, transition instructions are given to help you move smoothly from one exercise to the next. As you advance your routine, try to include these movements. Once you get practised at it, your whole routine should become one seamless movement with no pauses in between. It flows and has a meditative quality to it.

modifications

These are suggested to help you decrease, or occasionally increase, the intensity of the movement to suit your needs. Always read the Modifications first to see if they apply to you before attempting the main, more traditional version.

Only give your body the level of exercise that it requires. To get results, you need to be able to perform the exercise correctly, following every little detail, and to feel challenged without feeling that you are straining in any way. The challenge may come from any aspect of the exercise – the muscle strength required to perform it, your flexibility, your alignment, your stability, or your endurance.

injuries

Caution Boxes are included beside the exercises for anyone with injuries. The exercises are suitable for adults of all ages who are generally fit and well and suffering from no injuries or medical conditions. The **Caution Box** is only a basic guideline and cannot possibly cover every eventuality. If you have an injury or medical condition or are in any doubt as to whether a particular exercise is appropriate for your body, consult a doctor and a qualified instructor.

Pilates can be great for all sorts of remedial work, and for certain medical conditions, but only under the supervision of your doctor and a qualified instructor. See a professional first, and then ask for guidance on which exercises in this book are suitable or unsuitable for you.

If you find an exercise is putting a strain on your body, stop, re-read the instructions and check you are doing it correctly. Try again and if you still feel strain, and the suggested modification doesn't help, stop, and skip that exercise for now. As your strength and flexibility increase, try it again. Remember that some exercises may not be suitable for your body. Learn to listen to your body and only do what feels right for you.

listen to your body

Pilates should never be painful. An exercise may be hard work to perform, but it should never hurt, and you should never feel you are straining in any way.

backs

If you have no back injury or medical condition but feel a diffuse ache in your lower back while performing any of the exercises, this may be because you are not drawing in your abdominal muscles properly to protect your spine. Or it may be that your abdominal muscles are not yet strong enough to perform the movement. Try a modified version of the exercise, or reduce the number of repetitions until your abdominal muscles gain strength. If necessary, skip the exercise for the moment so you work without back tension. Exercises done when you are lying flat on your back, and therefore supported by the ground beneath you, are usually considered the safest ones for backs.

The exercises that are generally viewed as most challenging for bad backs, are ones that involve rolling, arching and twisting movements.

necks

If you have a weak neck, you should proceed with caution.

Remember to stay lifted using your abdominal muscles when performing a movement, and never lift with the neck itself. If your neck aches when lifting your head up while lying down, simply rest your head on your head rest for a while between repetitions, or perform the exercise with your head down. If it's more comfortable for you, exercise with a cushion or a rolled towel underneath your head to provide support until you grow stronger.

shoulders, elbows and wrists

If you have weak wrists, elbows or shoulders, you need to be extremely careful with weight-bearing exercises on your upper limbs. For shoulders and elbows, in particular, reduce the range of movement, working very slowly in a shortened range.

knees and ankles

If you have weak knees or ankles, you will need to be very careful with weight-bearing exercises on your lower limbs, such as those performed kneeling. You also need to avoid over-extending your knees or bending them in too tightly as this might aggravate them. Knee pain can sometimes be caused by improper leg and foot positioning, so pay particular attention to your alignment. Try to maintain a 'soft knee', bending it very slightly so it isn't locked while performing the movements.

hips

If you feel a slight ache in the hip while moving one or both of your legs in the air, and have no injury or medical condition, try bending the knee slightly.

self-assessment

As you work through each exercise, you need to monitor each movement. It is the attention to detail in Pilates which will change your body and your life.

beginner's pelvic tilt

Before you start your Pilates programme, try this exercise very slowly, then give yourself a body scan (see opposite).

If the exercise feels tough, or you feel any tension in your back, shoulders, chest or neck, don't come up so far from the floor. Just come up halfway until you grow stronger and more flexible.

1 Lie on your back with your knees bent at a 90-degree angle, feet parallel and hip-width apart. Your arms reach long by your sides with your palms facing down. Place your head on your book and draw your chin down slightly to ensure that the back of your neck is long (see page 26). Breathe laterally (see page 22), **inhaling** slowly and gently through the nose.

2 **Exhale**, engaging your pelvic floor and drawing in your abdominals (see page 23) as you peel your spine off the mat one vertebra at a time (see page 25) so that your hips curl up towards the ceiling. Press through your feet as you start to lift off, curling up as far as your body can go comfortably with the abdominals still engaged.

caution

● Proceed only under supervision if you have any back injuries or disc problems.

precision points

✗ Don't allow your knees to fall any further apart.

✗ Don't tense your neck, shoulders and chest. Keep the back of your neck long.

caution

● Proceed only under supervision if you have any back injuries or disc problems.

4 **Exhale**, drawing in the abdominals as you use them to roll down through your spine, lowering one vertebra at a time, leaving your arms behind you. *Imagine your spine softening and melting into the mat as you roll down.*

5 **Inhale**, lowering your arms to your sides. Repeat Steps 2–5 for required repetitions.

Transition: Bring your feet and knees together for the Small Hip Roll (see page 42), or lift your knees one at a time up towards your chest for the Side-to-Side (see page 74).

modifications

If the exercise feels tough, or you feel any tension in your back, shoulders, chest or neck, just come up half-way until you grow stronger and more flexible.

If you have shoulder problems, it may feel more comfortable to raise your arms to the ceiling rather than overhead, or just keep them on the floor. Keep the shoulder blades down into the back in both cases.

✓ **Try to isolate the vertebrae more each time you repeat the exercise.**

✓ **Bring your tailbone down onto the mat last: take care not to lower your bottom to the floor before you have rolled through each vertebra in your lower back.**

✓ **Relax the buttocks and be careful not to arch your lower back.**

small hip roll

body benefits

- strengthens and lengthens the abdominal muscles

- releases tension stored in the back and neck

- once the back and neck are freed up, posture immediately improves

repetitions: 10 each side, alternating sides

2 **Inhale**, rolling the knees to one side while pressing your opposite hand gently down on the hip to keep your hips and buttocks glued to the floor. You will not be able to go very far.

1 Lie on your back, with your knees bent at a 90-degree angle and feet together. Place your hands on your hips. Keep the back and the neck long.

precision points

✘ Don't allow your knees to fall apart.

✘ Don't twist your body.

caution

● This exercise is safe for most back injuries but always check with your doctor if you have any kind of back problem.

3 **Exhale**, drawing in the abdominals to return the knees to the centre. *Imagine your thighs are made of lead so that you really have to use your abdominal muscles to swing your knees back to centre each time.*

4 **Inhale** to take the knees over to the other side, while pressing gently down on the hip with the opposite hand.

5 **Exhale**, drawing in the abdominals again to return the knees to the centre.

Transition: Take the feet a little wider than hip-width apart for the Hip Roll (see page 44).

modifications

If your back is very stiff, don't take the knees as far over. Keep the movement very small at first.

✓ Be careful not to take your knees over too far, or your back, hips and bottom will lift.

✓ Keep your knees tightly together throughout.

✓ Roll straight from side to side with no twisting.

hip roll

body benefits

- strengthens the abdominal muscles

- stretches the hip flexors and lower back

- releases tension in the upper spine

- great for people with stiff shoulders, backs or necks

- once upper body tension is reduced, breathing improves

repetitions: 10 each side, alternating sides

modifications

If you feel tension in your lower back, don't take your knees over so far. If it still feels uncomfortable, just stick to the Small Hip Roll (see page 42) until you become stronger and more flexible.

If placing your hands behind your head is uncomfortable, reach the arms long by your sides with the palms facing down instead.

1 Lie on your back with your knees bent at a 90-degree angle and your feet slightly wider than hip-width apart. Your neck is long and your spine relaxed. Bend your arms and place both hands beneath your head, elbows wide. **Inhale**.

precision points

✗ Don't twist so far that your shoulder blades lift off the mat.

caution

● Omit this exercise if you have a bad neck or back injury.

2 **Exhale**, drawing in the abdominals, as you roll your knees towards the floor. The soles of your feet will come off the mat. As you stretch, let your head roll in the opposite direction to your knees so that you feel a stretch through your body. **Inhale** and rest in this position.

3 **Exhale**, drawing in the abdominals, to roll your knees all the way over to the other side. Let your head roll in the opposite direction. Imagine your lower abdominal muscles sinking down through your spine towards the floor. **Inhale** and rest in this position. Alternate smoothly from side to side.

Transition: Return to Step 1 position and move feet back to hip-width apart for the Chest Lift.

✓ Make sure your shoulder blades stay glued to the mat throughout.

✓ Only move when you are exhaling. Remain still as you inhale.

✓ Try to think of relaxing the fronts of your thighs as you move, and use the hollowing of the abdominals to initiate swinging the knees from one side to the other.

chest lift

body benefits

- strengthens the abdominal muscles for a firmer, flatter stomach

- highlights shoulder stabilization and neutral spine position

repetitions: 6–10

modifications

If your abdominal muscles start to quiver or pop out as you roll up, don't come up so high for the moment.

1 Lie on your back with your knees bent, feet and knees hip-width apart. Bend your arms to fold your hands behind your head, fingers interlaced and elbows out to the side. Check you are in neutral spine position. **Inhale**.

precision points

✗ Don't let your shoulder blades lift.

✗ Don't come out of your neutral spine position.

1 2 3

caution

● Proceed only under supervision if you have a back or neck injury.

2 **Exhale**, drawing in the abdominals, to roll your head and shoulders off the mat. As you roll up, slide your shoulder blades down into your back to keep the tops of your shoulders away from your ears. Keep your chin towards your chest with only a small space in between. *Imagine you are gently holding a peach under your chin.* **Inhale** and remain perfectly still in this lifted position.

3 **Exhale**, drawing in the abdominals to roll your head and shoulders back on to the mat.

Transition: Leave one arm behind your head and cross your other arm over to your opposite hip bone for the Oblique Reaches (see page 48), or take both arms by your sides and lift your knees towards your chest, one leg at a time, to prepare for The Hundred (see page 106).

✓Watch that the shoulder blades stay down into the back throughout to maintain good shoulder stabilization.

✓Make sure your abdominal muscles keep drawing in so they don't pop out as you roll up. There should be no tension in the back.

✓Support the weight of your head in your hands so there is no tension in the neck.

oblique reaches

body benefits

- strengthens the abdominal muscles (internal and external oblique muscles in particular, hence the name)

- trims the waist

repetitions: 6–10 each side

modifications

If you can't maintain neutral spine, and find you are tucking under and pressing your lower back into the mat, don't come up so high.

1 Lie on your back with your knees bent, feet hip-width apart. Bend one arm to fold one hand behind the head. The other hand rests on the opposite hipbone. **Inhale**.

precision points

✗ Don't let your tailbone lift off the floor to come out of neutral spine.

✗ Don't twist from your shoulders. Twist from your ribcage instead.

caution

● Proceed only under supervision if you have a neck or back injury.

2 **Exhale**, drawing in the abdominals to cross your arm over your body, stretching diagonally towards the outside of your opposite knee. Your palm faces down. Stay in neutral position, rotating your lower ribcage over to the side rather than just twisting the shoulders. *To stay in neutral, imagine there is an egg lying under your waist in the gentle curve of your back. As you twist over, be careful not to flatten your lower back and crush it.* Shoulder blades stay down into your back throughout.

3 **Inhale** and roll back down to Step 1 position keeping the stomach muscles engaged. Repeat Steps 2–3 for required repetitions.

Transition: Take both arms up to the ceiling for the Chest Opener (see page 50).

✓ **Lift both shoulders forward, but keep both shoulder blades down into the back as you move.**

✓ **Ensure the knees don't roll any wider apart.**

✓ **Relax your head in your hand so there is no tension in the neck.**

chest opener

body benefits

- opens the chest and counteracts rounded shoulders

- releases neck and shoulder tension and stiffness in the upper and mid-back

- strengthens and tones the chest and arms

repetitions: 6–10

modifications

If your shoulders are very tight, decrease the range of movement to begin with and just open the arms half-way.

1 Lie on your back with your knees bent at a 90-degree angle, feet hip-width apart. Make sure you are in neutral spine with your neck and shoulders relaxed. Lift both arms to the ceiling, shoulder-width apart, with your palms facing each other. Keep the arms straight without locking your elbows. Your hands should be level with your sternum.

precision points

✗ Don't bend your arms.

✗ Don't let your ribs stick out or arch your back as you open your arms.

caution

● Proceed with caution if you are prone to shoulder dislocation.

2 **Inhale** as you slowly open your arms straight out to the sides without bending them. Slide your shoulder blades down into your back as the arms open. *Imagine you are painting the arc of a rainbow beginning at the centre and working your way outwards to each end.*

3 **Exhale**, drawing in the abdominals, to return your arms to the starting position, using your chest muscles to perform the movement.

Transition: Turn your palms away from you to prepare for the Arm Splits (see page 52).

✓ Open your arms to a T-position. Don't allow your arms to move up to the top of your shoulders or to chin level as this can create tension.

✓ Keep your shoulder blades down into your back as you open your arms.

arm splits

body benefits

- strengthens and tones the back, chest and arm muscles

- releases tension in the neck, shoulders and upper back

- stretches the chest muscles to counteract round shoulders.

repetitions: 6–10 each way

2 **Exhale**, drawing in the abdominals, and split one arm in each direction so that your upper arm moves towards ear level, while you take your lower arm to hip level. Make sure your shoulder blades slide down into your back as you move, keeping the tops of your shoulders away from your ears. *Imagine your arms opening and closing like scissors.*

1 Lie on your back with your knees bent at a 90-degree angle, feet hip-width apart. Reach your arms up to the ceiling. Your arms are straight without locking your elbows, with your palms facing away from you. **Inhale**.

precision points

✗ Don't bend your arms or lift your shoulders towards your ears.

✗ Don't arch your back or lift your ribcage as you move.

caution

● If you have a recent shoulder injury, check with your doctor first, and go slowly and carefully on this one.

3 **Inhale** to return your arms to the starting position.

4 **Exhale**, drawing in the abdominals, and split the arms in the opposite direction.

modifications

If your shoulders are very tight, or the movement is uncomfortable, try reducing the range of movement and just take your arms half-way in each direction until you grow more flexible.

5 **Inhale** to return your arms to the ceiling.

Transition: Take your arms to your sides, straighten your legs out and roll on to your side for the Double Leg Lift (see page 54). Or take your arms to your sides, roll onto your side and press yourself up with your hands to come to a sitting position for the Roll Down (see page 76).

✓ Only take your upper arm back as far as you can while ensuring your shoulder blades stay down into your back and that your elbow doesn't bend.

✓ Go for quality of movement rather than trying to force your arm too low so that the tops of your shoulders lift up, and your forearm bends.

double leg lift

body benefits

- strengthens the abdominal muscles

- trims the waist

- firms the inner thighs

repetitions: 6–10 each side

modifications

If this position feels uncomfortable for your neck and shoulders, bend your lower arm slightly and place a cushion between your upper arm and head.

If you find it difficult to stop your hips from rolling, lie on your side with your back against a wall to begin with to ensure your hips and shoulders stay square.

1 Lie on your side with one hip carefully stacked on top of the other. Your ear, the middle of your shoulder, your hip and ankle should all be in a straight line. Your feet are pointing down.

Your upper arm rests on the floor in front of you, your lower arm stretches out above your head, palm up, your head resting on your arm. Now take your legs slightly further forward. **Inhale**.

precision points

✗ Don't roll your hips or shoulders forwards.

✗ Don't collapse at the waist.

① ② ③

caution

● Proceed only under supervision if you have a back injury.

2 **Exhale**, drawing in the abdominals to stabilize your body, and lift both straight legs off the mat – about 10 cm (4 in) squeezing your inner thighs together as you lift, and stretching your legs away from you. *Imagine your inner thighs have been stuck together with glue so they move as a single unit.* Hold for a count of three.

3 **Inhale** as you slowly lower both legs down.

Transition: Bend your lower leg forwards for the Outer Thigh Lift (see page 56), or turn your legs out for the Side Kick (see page 118). To save you switching back and forth from one side to the other while you complete the side-lying leg series that follows, you can perform all the side-lying exercises on one side before rolling over to your other side to repeat them in order on the other side.

✓Keep your torso still. Don't arch your lower back or twist your pelvis or shoulders.

✓Be careful not to shorten your waist. If you stretch your legs away from you, there should be a small gap between your waist and the mat – maintain this throughout.

✓Squeeze your inner thighs together as you lift.

outer thigh lift

body benefits

- tones the outer thigh muscles to reduce saddlebags and create slimmer thighs

- strengthens the buttock muscles

- stretches the leg muscles all the way from your bottom right down to your ankles

repetitions: 6–10 each side

modifications

If you find it uncomfortable lying on your straight arm, bend the arm slightly and place a cushion under your head.

If you find it difficult to get a good alignment, lie with your back against a wall to ensure your hips and shoulders stay square.

1 Lie on your side with one hip carefully stacked on top of the other. Your ear, the middle of your shoulder, your hip and ankle should all be in a straight line. Your feet are pointing down. Your upper arm rests on the floor in front of you, the lower arm stretches out above your head, palm up, your head resting on your arm. Bend your lower leg forwards to give a little more support. Reach your upper leg away from you without moving your hips, and flex your foot. Turn the thigh of the upper leg inward in the hip socket so that the leg is slightly internally rotated, without actually moving the hip itself. **Inhale**.

precision points

✗ Don't allow the small of your waist to collapse into the floor.

✗ Don't allow your hip to roll forwards as you lift your top leg to hip height.

2 **Exhale**, drawing in the abdominals to keep your body stable and squeezing your buttock muscles gently together, stretch the upper leg away from you, as you lift it level with the hip. Lengthen your waist and really reach your upper leg away from you, keeping the internal rotation, pushing through the heel of your foot as you lift. *Imagine you are trying to touch the wall opposite you with your heel.*

3 **Inhale** and lower your leg to your starting position.

Transition: Straighten your lower leg and cross your upper leg over it for the Inner Thigh Lift (see page 58).

✓ Your lower ribs should remain still and not push forwards.

✓ The alignment of your body is vital in this exercise. Keep your body in a straight line with your hips facing forwards. Don't let them roll forwards or backwards as you move.

✓ Keep the foot flexed throughout. If you have internally rotated your thigh in the hip socket correctly, your heel will be slightly higher than your toes.

inner thigh lift

body benefits

- strengthens and firms the inner thigh muscles

repetitions: 6–10 each side

2 **Exhale**, drawing in the abdominals, and stretch your lower leg away from you as you slowly lift the heel about 15 cm (6 in) off the mat. Make sure you keep your lower knee facing forwards throughout and that your hips don't move. *Imagine that you are trying to touch the wall opposite you with your heel.*

1 Lie on your side with one hip carefully stacked on top of the other. Your ear, the middle of your shoulder, your hip and ankle should all be in a straight line. Your feet are pointing down. Your upper arm rests on the floor in front of you, your lower arm stretches out above your head, palm up, your head resting on your arm. Bring your top leg in front of you so that the foot of your upper leg rests on the floor keeping the leg straight and one hip stacked on top of the other. Your lower leg remains straight underneath it. **Inhale**.

precision points

✗ Don't bend your leg.

✗ Don't allow your hips to roll forwards or back.

3

Inhale as you lower your leg to the mat.

Transition: After completing the inner thigh lift on both sides, roll onto your front for the Hamstring Lift (see page 60), or the Single Leg Kick (see page 120).

modifications

If you find this uncomfortable for your shoulders, bend your lower arm slightly and rest a cushion on top of your arm on which to rest your head.

If it is difficult to keep your back and hips stable, or your top leg straight, perform this exercise with your back against a wall, bend your top leg and rest it on two pillows to stabilize your hips.

To ensure that your hip doesn't move and that you concentrate the work on the inner thigh, place your upper hand just below your hip and gently press down towards the mat.

✓ Make sure that the hip, knee and foot of the lower leg face forwards.

✓ Keep your torso still.

✓ Think of pushing through the heel of your lower foot to lengthen the leg away from you as you lift. You should feel the inner thigh working to lift your leg up.

✓ Keep the whole movement slow and smooth.

hamstring lift

body benefits

- lifts and tones the buttocks

- strengthens the hamstring muscles in the back of the thighs

- stretches the legs for a more stream-lined appearance

repetitions: 6–10 on each leg

1 Lie on your front with your legs stretched away from you, feet together. Bend your elbows and place your hands one on top of the other under your forehead. Press your pubic bone gently towards the mat to lengthen your lower back. **Inhale**.

precision points

✗ Don't lift your shoulders.

✗ Don't lift your hips along with your leg.

1 2 3

2 **Exhale**, drawing in the abdominals, and lift one leg off the mat, stretching the leg along its length from where it meets the buttock all the way down to the heel. Hold for a count of six. *Imagine your leg is like a piece of sticky toffee, growing thinner and thinner as you stretch it in opposite directions.*

3 **Inhale** and lower your leg.

Transition: Place your arms by your sides and rest your forehead on the head rest for the Arrow (see page 62).

✓ To protect your lower back, ensure you keep the abdominals pulled in as you lift so that your lower abdomen pulls away from the floor.

✓ Think of pushing your heel away from you to touch the wall opposite, to really lengthen the leg.

✓ Lengthen the back of your neck and relax your shoulders throughout.

arrow

body benefits

- back and abdominal muscles are strengthened and in time this will help with lower back aches and pains

- helps to improve shoulder stabilization

repetitions: 6–10

2 **Exhale**, drawing in the abdominals, as you lift your palms towards the ceiling, sliding your shoulder blades down your back towards your hips and lifting your sternum and head and shoulders off the mat. Hold this position for a count of three. *Imagine your body as a streamlined arrow.* Press the crown of your head away from you to keep the back of your neck lengthened and to stretch your spine. At the same time, reach your fingertips in the opposite direction.

1 Lie face down on the mat with your arms by your sides, palms up and fingers pointing towards your feet.

Press your pubic bone gently into the mat to keep your lower back long. **Inhale**.

precision points

✗ Don't lift your legs.

✗ Don't crunch the back of the neck or look forwards instead of down at the mat.

3 **Inhale** and lower your body down.

Transition: Press your palms down on the mat in front of you and push yourself back so that

your bottom rests on your heels for the Rest Position (see below).

rest position

body benefits

● a great opportunity to cool down towards the end of your session and to stretch your lower back

1 From the Arrow position draw your body back so that you are sitting back on

your heels with your arms stretched out in front of you. Rest here for about 30 seconds.

Transition: Slowly roll back up to a kneeling position coming up one vertebra at a time. Sit

on the mat and then roll down onto your back for the Hamstring Stretch (see page 64).

✓ Think of this more as a long stretch than a lift. Don't bring your arms or your body too high off the floor. When your arms lift, the palms should come just above the top of your

buttocks. Your head lifts about 10 cm (4 in) off the mat. You are then resting on your ribs, pubic bone hipbones and legs.

✓ Keep your abdominals lifted throughout to support your spine.

✓ Make sure you lengthen through the back of your neck throughout.

hamstring stretch

body benefits

- lengthens the hamstring muscles in the back of the thighs

- helps to release a tight lower back

1 Lie on your back with your knees bent and feet hip-width apart. Raise one leg and place your hands behind your thigh to support it. **Inhale**, making sure your tailbone is down on the mat.

2 **Exhale**, drawing in the abdominals, as you stretch your raised leg up towards the ceiling using your hands to support your leg as it extends. Flex the foot. Hold this for about 30 seconds. Repeat on the other leg.

modifications

If this position is uncomfortable for you, use a belt or dressing gown cord to support your foot.

If you have fairly flexible hamstrings, you can stretch the leg, which isn't supported by your hands away from you along the mat so that the leg lies straight rather than bent.

precision points

✗ Don't get carried away with this stretch. Ensure you keep your tailbone down throughout so that the pelvis doesn't tilt even if this means not taking the leg as high.

✓ Think of stretching your raised leg in two directions: the heel up towards the ceiling, but also the other end of the leg, near the buttocks, down into the floor.

✓ Remember to keep your shoulders relaxed and your head on the head rest.

quadriceps stretch

body benefits

● lengthens the quadriceps muscles in the front of the thighs

caution

● Proceed with caution if you have problem knees and omit this exercise if it feels uncomfortable.

1 Lie on your side in a straight line, with your lower arm above your head, palm up, with the head resting on your arm. Bend your lower leg forwards to support you. The higher up you can place this bent leg, the better the muscles will stretch. **Inhale**.

2 **Exhale**, drawing in the abdominals, and reach down to take hold of the ankle of your upper leg and draw it behind you towards your buttocks. You will feel your quadriceps muscle in the front of your thigh stretching. Hold the stretch for 30 seconds keeping your abdominal muscles engaged. Roll over onto your other side and repeat.

precision points

✗ Don't arch your back and don't roll your body forwards or backwards.

✓ Gently push your hips forward a little to increase the stretch.

buttock stretch

body benefits

● stretches the buttock muscles

● helps to release a tight lower back

1 Lie down on your back with one knee bent at a 90-degree angle. Cross your other leg over and place the ankle just above the knee. Hold this ankle while keeping your head on the floor. **Inhale**.

precision points

✗ Don't twist your hips.

✗ Don't lift your shoulders or your tailbone.

caution

● Proceed only under supervision if you have a back or neck injury.

4 **Inhale**, keeping the abdominals engaged, as you take your knees over to the other side, rolling your head in the opposite direction.

5 **Exhale**, drawing in the abdominals to return to centre.

Transition: Place the feet back on to the mat, with the knees bent at a 90-degree angle, and feet hip-width apart. Take the arms behind the head for the Chest Lift (see page 46).

modifications

If you feel any tension in your lower back, or this exercises feels too much for your abdominal muscles, replace it with both the Small Hip Roll (see page 42) and the Hip Roll (see page 44) exercises in Level 1 until your body grows stronger.

✓ Relax your neck, chest and shoulders

✓ Keep your shoulder blades down on the mat throughout.

✓ Press your palms into the mat for extra stability.

✓ Make sure you take your knees and feet directly over to the side without twisting your hips.

✓ Your knees and feet should move over to the side as a single unit.

roll down

body benefits

- strengthens the abdominal muscles

- stretches the back to improve flexibility

- encourages good spinal articulation

repetitions: 3–5

2 **Exhale**, drawing in the abdominals, and curl your tailbone under you, aiming your lower back for the mat so that your spine forms a C-shaped curve. As you **continue to exhale**, keep drawing in the abdominals and try to increase the C-curve by rolling your spine down one vertebra at a time. Roll as far down as your arms will allow without your hands coming away from your thighs. Your shoulder blades stay down into your back. **Inhale** and rest in the C-curve position.

1 Sit up tall with a straight back, with your knees bent at a 90-degree angle and feet hip-width apart. Place your feet as flat as possible. Place your hands around the back of your thighs and lift your elbows wide. **Inhale**.

precision points

✗ Don't allow your ribs to lift or your abdominals to bulge.

✗ Don't straighten your back as you move; it should be curved.

caution

● Omit this exercise if you feel any tension in your lower back.

● Hold your legs lightly if you have weak wrists, elbows or shoulders.

3 **Exhale**, drawing in the abdominals deeper and deeper, to curl back up one vertebra at a time, keeping the C-curve all the way up until your shoulders are above your hips. *Imagine your abdominals are being drawn back towards your spine by a supermagnetic force.*

4 **Inhale** and sit up tall again with a straight back.

Transition: Lower yourself down to the mat with your arms by your sides for the Single Leg Circles (see page 78).

modifications

Keep your feet flat on the mat, if possible. If this is uncomfortable, lift the toes but keep your heels on the mat.

✓ **Be careful not to lean your body back. Instead, use your abdominals so the movement begins from the base of your spine.**

✓ **Keep the abdominal muscles drawing in to curve your lower back.**

✓ **Keep your shoulder blades down into your back and your elbows lifted.**

single leg circles

body benefits

- increases strength and flexibility in the hips

- lengthens the back of the thighs

- strengthens the inner thighs

- stretches and strengthens the outer thighs

- firms the buttocks

repetitions: 5 circles in each direction with one leg, 5 circles in each direction with the other leg.

1 Lie on your back with your knees bent at a 90-degree angle, feet hip-width apart. Place your arms by your sides, pressing your palms down into the mat for support. Ensure that the back of your neck is lengthened and your shoulders down and relaxed. Lift one straight leg up to the ceiling, turning out the leg (see page 27) by engaging the lower buttock muscles to rotate the thigh outwards in the hip socket. Your inner thigh also engages. Point your toe. Your other leg remains bent with the foot firmly planted on the mat.

caution

● Proceed only under supervision if you have a back injury.

● If you experience any clicking in your hip, try bending your knee slightly, and reducing the size of the circle.

2 **Inhale** as you cross your leg over your body without letting your hips lift off the mat.

3 **Exhale**, drawing in the abdominals, as you sweep your leg in a circle down towards the mid-line of your body.

single leg circles cont.

4 Keep **exhaling** as you continue the circle round to the other side of your body.

5 Then circle your leg back up to its starting position in the centre, still **exhaling**. *Imagine you are painting a small circle in the air, using your big toe as the paintbrush.* Control the movement with your abdominals so that your torso and your bent leg stay completely still throughout. Repeat 5 times.

precision points

✗ **Don't lift the pelvis.**

✗ **Don't crunch the neck and shoulders.**

6 Reverse the circle by **inhaling** to take your leg over to the side away from your body. **Exhale** as you take the leg down, around and back to the centre. Repeat 5 times.

Transition: Place both feet back on the mat, knees bent, then roll on to one side and push yourself up with your hands to come up to sitting for Rolling Like a Ball (see page 82).

Or, if you are able, lower your raised leg, take your arms above your head and perform a Roll-up (see page 108) to bring you up to sitting position for Rolling Like a Ball.

modifications

If you have a tight lower back and hamstrings, holding the position may feel a little difficult. If you are unable to keep both hips down on the mat while straightening the leg to the ceiling, bend the knee slightly until you are able to straighten the leg out comfortably.

Once you can perform the Single Leg Circles whilst keeping your torso stable when the lower knee is bent, you can challenge yourself further by straightening this leg along the mat.

Once you can perform the movement while keeping your torso completely stable, challenge yourself further by increasing the size of the circle without sacrificing your core stability.

✓ Ensure that your body remains still while you circle your leg in your hip joint so that you don't roll off to one side and your back does not arch.

✓ In order to stop your quadriceps from doing all the work, keep your thigh turned out slightly in the hip and think of using your buttock to help make the movement.

✓ Your toes reach for the ceiling as you circle to keep your leg completely straight.

✓ The emphasis of this movement is on the 'upswing'.

rolling like a ball

body benefits

- strengthens the abdominals

- massages the spine and improves spinal flexibility

- improves balance and control

repetitions: 6–10

2 **Inhale** as you roll back on the mat to the base of your shoulder blades, keeping your rounded shape. Feel your spine roll back on to the mat one vertebra at a time so that you end up with your bottom towards the ceiling. *Imagine you are running up the scale on a piano as you try to feel each vertebra connecting with the mat.*

1 Sit near the front of your mat with your feet together and knees bent. Take hold of one ankle in each hand with elbows wide to the sides. Pull your feet close to your buttocks and roll your head down towards your knees. Open your knees slightly. Rock back fractionally so that your back is rounded and you are balancing on your tailbone with your feet just lifted off the floor. You want to keep this rounded ball shape throughout.

precision points

✗

✗ Don't move your feet away from your buttocks. Keep a tight ball shape.

✗ Don't let your head touch the mat

caution

● Proceed only under supervision if you have a back injury.

● Omit if you have a severe scoliosis.

3 **Exhale**, drawing in the abdominals, to roll back up to your starting position so that you are balancing on your tailbone again, keeping a rounded spine. Your feet hover just above the ground. Keep your shoulder blades down into your back throughout.

Transition: From sitting, roll down to the mat one vertebra at a time, and draw the knees towards the chest to prepare for the Beginner's Double Leg Stretch (see page 84).

modifications

Don't worry if you can't roll all the way back up initially, just roll up as high as you can and continue to practice.

If the exercise feels very difficult, place one hand behind each thigh instead, elbows wide. Still keep the feet together, the knees slightly open, and the lower back curved. Try rolling in this position.

✓ **Keep your shoulders relaxed and down through-out. Don't let them creep up around your ears.**

✓ **Keep your head towards your knees, especially when rolling up.**

✓ **Once you've found the movement, try not to use too much momentum. Instead use your abdominal strength to get you back up.**

✓ **Keep your lower back curved throughout, so that you don't straighten your back at the balance point, in particular.**

beginner's double leg stretch

body benefits

- strengthens the abdominals

- strengthens the leg muscles

repetitions: 6–10

2 Continue this exhalation as you straighten your legs towards the ceiling, pointing your toes. *Imagine your back is glued to the floor.*

1 Lie on your back with your knees bent and shins parallel to the floor; your knees are at a 90-degree angle to your torso. Interlace your fingers and place your hands behind your head with your head resting on the mat. Your elbows are wide but should just be within your peripheral vision. **Inhale**, then **exhale** slowly, drawing in your abdominals, and rolling your head and shoulders off the mat, hinging at the breastbone as you slide your shoulderblades down your back.

precision points

✗ Don't allow your elbows to fall inwards.

✗ Don't arch your back.

caution

● Proceed only under supervision if you have a neck or back injury.

3 **Inhale** and rebend your knees with your abdominal muscles still engaged.

4 **Exhale**, drawing in the abdominals, as you roll your head back onto the mat.

Transition: Rest both hands lightly on one knee for the Single Leg Stretch (see page 86).

modifications

If you can't fully straighten your legs to the ceiling, straighten them as far as you can, and perform the exercise with the legs slightly bent.

Once you are comfortable performing the exercise with the legs straight, you can begin to lower your straight legs to an angle of 45 degrees. If your back starts to arch off the mat, you have taken the legs too low.

✓ Let your head be heavy in your hands. Use your abdominals to lift so there is no strain in the neck.

✓ Keep the elbows wide and the shoulders relaxed.

✓ Keep your back flat on the mat throughout.

single leg stretch

body benefits

- tones the abdominal muscles

- trims the waist

- encourages good body alignment

repetitions: 6–10 each side, alternating legs

3 **Exhale**, drawing in the abdominals as you straighten one leg at a 45-degree angle. Your torso and your other leg, supported by your two hands, don't move. You are now in the starting position. *Imagine your torso is frozen in ice and cannot move.* **Inhale**.

2 **Inhale**, keeping the abdominals engaged, and roll your head and shoulders off the mat, sliding your shoulder blades down into your back.

1 Lie on your back with your knees bent and shins parallel to the mat. Place one hand on the inside of your opposite knee. The other hand reaches down the outside of your leg, towards your ankle. Knees are close together. The elbows are wide. **Inhale**, then **exhale**, drawing in the abdominals.

precision points

✗ **Don't twist your shoulders and hips.**

✗ **Don't drop your bent leg.**

4 Without changing the position of your torso, **exhale** and draw in the abdominals as you switch legs, bending your straight leg in, switching your hands over to that leg, while straightening your other leg out to 45 degrees. Continue to switch legs on each exhalation for the required number of repetitions. Between exhalations, there is the tiniest of in-breaths, almost a 'sniff'. The focus is on the out-breath as you bend one leg in and straighten the other.

Transition: Take the hands behind the head for the Beginner's Criss-Cross (see page 114). Or roll over on to one side and press yourself up to sitting with your hands to prepare for the Spine Stretch Forwards (see page 88).

modifications

If you find it difficult to keep your back flat on the mat, try straightening your leg towards the ceiling instead. As your strength improves, bring your leg to a lower angle.

If you feel tension in the neck, perform the leg movements with both hands behind your head, supporting the weight of your head with your hands.

If this still feels tough, rest your head and shoulders on the head rest throughout, placing both hands on one knee.

If your knee aches, hold under the knee instead and take the exercise at a slower pace so there is no pain, or omit it entirely.

✓ **Keep your back flat on the mat throughout and your shoulder blades down.**

✓ **Pay attention to your hand positions as this keeps you aligned correctly.**

✓ **Keep your torso and bent leg completely still as you lengthen the other leg away.**

✓ **Watch that your bent leg stays at a 90-degree angle and that your foot and calf don't start to flop towards the floor.**

spine stretch forwards

body benefits

- works the abdominal muscles

- a great stretch for the lower back

- improves spinal flexibility

- stretches the back of the legs

- improves sitting posture

repetitions: 3–5

2 **Exhale**, drawing in the abdominals, and round your spine forwards one vertebra at a time. Keep rolling forwards until your spine forms a letter C-shaped curve. *Imagine your straight back is against a wall. Lower your head, then peel your* *upper back off the wall, followed by your mid-back and finally your lower back.* Try to resist the stretch by drawing in your abdominals as you round forwards, stretching your lower back further behind you. Your head should end up just above your arms, following the line of the C-shaped curve.

1 Sit up tall with your legs straight, hip-width apart, and your feet flexed so that your toes point to the ceiling. Lift your arms parallel to your legs at shoulder height, ensuring the shoulder blades are relaxed down into your back. **Inhale**.

precision points

✗ **Don't hold your arms too high, they should stay at shoulder height.**

✗ **Don't hold your back straight as you roll forwards.**

caution

● Proceed only under supervision if you have any kind of back injury.

● Proceed with caution if you have any stiffness in the lower back.

3 **Inhale**, then **exhale**, drawing in your abdominals as you reverse the movement. Roll back up your imaginary wall to your tall sitting position, one vertebra at a time, placing your lower back, then your mid- and then upper back, and finally your head. Keep pulling your abdominals in until you're sitting up really tall. Focus on lifting up out of your hips with a straight back.

Transition: Take your feet just wider than hip-width apart, and reach your arms out to the sides at shoulder height for the Saw (see page 90).

modifications

If the stretch behind your knees is too much, bend your knees slightly so the thigh muscles relax.

If the stretch is too much in your lower back, or you find it hard to sit up tall due to a tight lower back or hamstrings, bend your knees slightly and don't roll down as far. Gradually increase the range of movement as you grow more flexible.

✓ Keep the space between your ribcage and hips. Imagine you are stretching up and over a beach ball positioned between your legs so you don't collapse your torso as you roll.

✓ As you roll, keep your feet flexed and think of pushing through your heels to really feel the stretch in the backs of your legs.

✓ Watch that there is no tension in your neck throughout the stretch. Just let your head hang.

✓ Roll back up to sit tall, without leaning forwards or back, your shoulder blades down into your back, and reaching the crown of your head up to the ceiling.

saw

body benefits

- stretches the waist, hips and back of thighs

- improves spinal rotation

- helps to empty and cleanse the lungs

repetitions: 3–5 each side, alternating sides

3 **Exhale**, drawing in the abdominals, as you round forwards, reaching your front arm forwards and down, aiming for your little toe. *Imagine you are sawing off your little toe with your little finger.* The back hand sweeps back and lowers to line up with the front hand.

2 **Inhale** and slowly twist your upper body from the waist. Let the arms float with you until your forward arm is directly over your opposite leg. Lengthen your spine up as you twist, keeping your hips and legs glued to the mat.

1 Sit up tall, reaching up through the crown of your head to lengthen your spine up towards the ceiling. Reach your arms out straight to the sides, so that you can just see them within your peripheral vision, with the palms facing down. Your legs are straight, just wider than hip-width apart, with your feet flexed.

precision points

✗ Don't allow your hips to roll.

caution

● Omit this exercise if you have a back or neck injury.

4 **Inhale**, remaining on the diagonal as you roll, one vertebra at a time, back to sitting. Initiate this movement from your centre. As you come up, lift your arms until they are shoulder height and parallel to the floor.

5 **Exhale**, drawing in the abdominals, and twist from the waist back to centre and your Step 1 starting position. Repeat, twisting to the other side.

Transition: Bring your straight legs together for the Spine Twist (see page 92).

modifications

If the stretch is too much for the back of your knees, or if you find it hard to sit up straight, bend your knees slightly to give yourself extra lift.

✓Ensure that you twist from your waist, not from your shoulders or hips. Keep your hipbones facing forwards as you twist.

✓Your head rolls forwards with your body and your neck is relaxed.

✓Roll up through the spine to come back to sitting, don't straighten up with a flat back. Your head should be the last part to come up.

spine twist

body benefits

- stretches the spine

- lengthens the muscles in the back of the legs

- trims the waistline

- wrings stale air from your lungs

repetitions: 5 each side, alternating sides

2 **Exhale**, drawing in the abdominals, and twist to one side with a double pulse at the furthest point in the stretch. As you twist, keep your hips still and reach up through the crown of your head to lengthen your spine. **Exhale fully**. *Imagine your are wringing your spine as you twist, as you would wring water from a towel.*

1 Sit up tall with your arms stretched out to the sides. Your palms face down and your shoulder blades are down into your back throughout. Your arms should lie just within your peripheral vision. Your legs are straight with your thighs squeezed tightly together and your feet flexed so your toes point to the ceiling. **Inhale**.

precision points

✗ Don't twist from your shoulders or let your body fall forward.

✗ Don't allow your heel bones to come out of alignment.

caution

● Omit this exercise if you have back problems.

● If you have a delicate shoulder, only twist as far as you can without any pain.

3 **Inhale** to twist back to centre.

4 **Exhale**, drawing in the abdominals, as you twist to the other side with a double pulse. **Inhale** as you return to centre.

Transition: Roll on to one side in a straight line for the Double Leg Lift (see page 54). Or bend your knees and roll down one vertebra at a time so that you are lying on your back to prepare for the Corkscrew (see page 116).

modifications

If you feel too much stress on the backs of your legs, or you find you can't sit up with a straight spine, bend your knees slightly for more lift.

✓If you find one heel moves further forward than the other, you are incorrectly moving your hip.

✓Only twist from your waist, your hipbones remain facing forwards throughout.

✓Allow your head to follow the twist in your spine. Don't overturn the head.

plank

body benefits

- builds upper body strength in particular, but tones and strengthens the whole body

- strengthens back, chest, shoulders, back of thighs, buttocks, abdominal muscles and arms

repetitions: 3

2 Reach one leg back and place the ball of your foot on the floor, straightening your leg out and putting your weight on it.

1 Kneel on all fours with your hands directly underneath your shoulders. Keep your arms straight, but don't lock your elbows. Knees should be hip-width apart.

precision points

✗ Don't let your hips sink so the diagonal line is lost.

✗ Don't let your shoulders collapse.

caution

● Omit this exercise if you have a shoulder or elbow injury.

● Omit this exercise if you have weak hands or wrists.

3 Straighten your other leg out to join the first and place your weight evenly between the balls of your two feet. Your feet should be side by side with your legs pressed tightly together. Draw your abdominals up into the body to support the spine throughout. Your arms are straight with your shoulders pressed down away from your ears. Your body forms a plank – a straight line from your shoulders all the way down to your heels. *Imagine you are a rod of steel that cannot sag*. Hold this position for 2–4 breaths. Bend the knees to rest, then repeat twice more.

Transition: Bend the legs in and down to the floor to return to the kneeling position. Turn over and sit up tall with your legs stretched out in front of you to prepare for the Reverse Plank (see page 96).

modifications

If you are not yet strong enough to maintain the plank position, or you find it is placing strain on your wrists, omit this exercise for the moment.

✓Plant your hands and feet firmly into the mat.

✓Lengthen through the crown of your head to keep the back of your neck long. Your neck should be aligned with the rest of your spine. Look down.

✓Squeeze your thighs together and slightly engage your buttocks to maintain your 'rod of steel'.

✓To keep your pelvis aligned, think of tucking your pubic bone under slightly. Don't allow your bottom to lift or to sink.

reverse plank

body benefits

- challenges abdominal strength

- firms and strengthens the buttocks and back of thighs

- strengthens the upper torso

repetitions: 3

1 Sit up tall with your legs stretched out in front of you and your hands behind you, fingers pointing towards your body. Squeeze your inner thighs together throughout. **Inhale**.

precision points

✘ Don't allow your hips and shoulders to collapse.

✘ Don't throw your head back.

caution

● Omit this exercise if you have a shoulder or elbow injury.

● Omit this exercise if you have weak hands or wrists.

2 **Exhale**, drawing in the abdominals, and press your hips up to the ceiling to establish a reverse plank position. Engage your buttock muscles, and slide your shoulder blades down into your back to hold yourself in one long straight line from shoulders to feet. Look straight ahead. *Imagine you are a rod of steel and cannot sag.* Hold this position for 2–4 breaths. Lower your hips to the mat to rest and repeat twice more.

Transition: Slowly lower your hips and return to Step 1 position. Press your hands into the mat either side of you and lift yourself forwards so that you are sitting at the front of your mat to prepare for the Seal (see page 98).

modifications

If holding this position is uncomfortable on your hands and wrists, try turning your palms out so that your fingers point out to the sides.

If the above modification is still difficult for you, omit this exercise for the moment.

To start with, let your head be positioned so that your eyes look forwards. As you progress, try to keep your head and neck aligned with your spine.

✓ **Lengthen the crown of your head up to the ceiling to elongate the back of your neck.**

✓ **Slide your shoulder blades down into your back.**

✓ **Use your abdominals and engage your buttock muscles to keep your hips lifted.**

✓ **Heels remain on the mat even if your toes need to lift slightly.**

seal

body benefits

- fantastic spinal massage

- improves spinal flexibility

- strengthens the abdominal muscles

- improves balance and control

- a great cool-down exercise

repetitions: 5–10

1 Sit at the front of your mat with your knees bent towards your chest and heels together. Open your knees to shoulder width and thread your hands through the legs to hold the outside of your ankles.

Round your back and rock back a fraction so that your feet are just off the mat and you are balancing on your tailbone. Bring your chin slightly towards your chest.

precision points

✗ Don't lift your shoulders.

✗ Don't throw your head back and forth or roll on to your neck.

caution

● Omit this exercise if you have a bad neck or back injury.

● Proceed with caution if you have weak wrists or elbows.

2 **Inhale**, smoothly rolling backwards one vertebra at a time, until the base of your shoulder blades touch the mat and your bottom lifts towards the ceiling. Clap your heels together 3 times *like a seal clapping its flippers*, keeping your chin tucked towards your chest.

3 **Exhale**, drawing in your abdominals to roll back up to your balance point at the end of Step 1. Clap heels together again 3 times.

modifications

If it is difficult to rock back and forth, leave out the claps for now, and just focus on using your abdominals to roll each way. As you get stronger, just add the claps after the forwards movement. You can add the claps after the backwards movement later.

✓ **Focus on balancing at the beginning and end of the movement.**

✓ **Use your breath and control of your abdominals to bring you forwards and back. Try not to rely on momentum.**

✓ **Keep your shoulder blades down your back, and make sure your lower back is curved throughout.**

sure you are still taking all the Precision Points on board, and also to see if you now

need to graduate to a more challenging Modified version.

4
the hundred* p106

5
roll up* p108

6
single leg circles p78

10
beginner's criss-cross*
p114

11
spine stretch forwards p88

12
saw p90

16
side kick* p118

17
outer thigh lift p56

18
inner thigh lift p58

22
reverse plank p96

23
seal p98

the hundred

body benefits

- the ultimate abdominal strengthener

- strengthens upper back and chest muscles

- stimulates circulation

- builds stamina

3 Exhale, drawing in the abdominals a little deeper, and stretch your legs up towards the ceiling. Keep the inner thighs glued together. *Imagine a heavy weight bearing down on your stomach as it sinks down towards the floor.* Look towards your navel.

2 Inhale, keeping the abdominals engaged and initiating from them to roll your head and shoulders off the mat, hinging forward from the sternum. Stretch your arms away from you past your hips, keeping your shoulder blades down and your neck relaxed.

1 Lie on your back with your knees bent and your arms by your sides, palms down. Bend your knees in towards your chest. Lengthen the back of your neck and slide your shoulder blades down into your back. **Inhale**, then **exhale**, drawing in the abdominals.

precision points

✗

✗ Don't lift your back too high off the mat.

✗ Don't allow your shoulders to lift up towards your ears.

caution

● This is a tough exercise. If you feel any pain in your lower back, omit this exercise. If you feel tension in the lower back even when trying the modified version, omit this exercise until you can perform the exercise without arching your back or your abdominal muscles popping out.

4 Begin pumping your arms briskly up and down initiating from underneath the shoulder blades.

Inhale for 5 pumps and **exhale** for 5 pumps. Pump 100 times (i.e. 10 full breath cycles).

Transition: Draw your knees in towards your chest, rolling your head and shoulders down to prepare for the Roll Up (see page 108).

modifications

You may not be able to complete 100 pumps to start with. Begin with 50 and gradually increase the number of pumps each time you do the exercise.

If your back is arching or there is any

tension in your lower back, bend your knees while you pump. Start to lengthen your legs to a 90-degree angle when you are stronger.

When you can comfortably perform the exercise with

straight legs, lower your legs to increase the level of difficulty. Gradually advance to a 45-degree angle.

If you feel any tension in your neck, just lower your head down and rest for a

while before trying again. If you still feel tension, take your hands behind your head and support the weight of your head in your hands while you stay in your position for the 10 breath cycles.

✓**Keep your back flat on the mat and your shoulder blades down throughout.**

✓**Ensure there is no tension in your neck. Think of hinging your body forwards from your sternum, using your abdominals, not by pulling your neck forwards.**

✓**Keep the pumps small and brisk, no higher than mid-thigh level. Keep your arms close to your body.**

✓**Breathe gently in through your nose and out through your mouth.**

roll up

body benefits

- strengthens the abdominal muscles

- stretches the back to improve flexibility

- encourages good spinal articulation

- lengthens the muscles in the back of the thighs

repetitions: 3–5

2 **Inhale**, keeping the abdominals engaged, as you lift your arms forwards to roll your head and shoulders off the mat, hinging forward from the sternum. Make sure your shoulder blades are down and the base of your shoulder blades still touching the mat.

1 Lie on your back with your knees bent, feet and knees together. Reach your arms overhead, just above the level of your ears. Squeeze your inner thighs together. **Inhale**, then **exhale**, drawing in the abdominals.

caution

● Omit this exercise if you have any kind of back injury.

3 **Exhale**, drawing in the abdominals as you curl your body off the mat, peeling your spine off it one vertebra at a time. Try to create a letter C-shaped curve with your spine as you come up, pulling your abdominals deeper and deeper in the higher you come.

4 Keep rolling forwards as you continue to **exhale**, rounding over with your arms parallel to the mat and your fingers in line with your ankles. Once your fingers reach past your knees straighten your legs with feet flexed as you continue to come forwards. *Imagine you are rolling up and over a beach ball placed on your thighs.* Your will probably feel the stretch in the back of your thighs.

roll up cont.

6 **Exhale**, drawing in the abdominals, and continue this flowing movement to roll your spine back down to the mat one vertebra at a time. Keep the C-shaped curve of your back throughout. You will feel your pelvis sliding underneath you as you roll back, and your shoulder blades stay down into your back. You are in Step 3 position again.

5 Reverse the movement. **Inhale** as you start to roll back until your shoulders are level with your hips. Slowly rebend your knees.

precision points

✗

✗ Don't flatten your back; it should be in a C-shaped curve.

✗ Don't let your abdominal muscles pop out as you roll up.

7 Once your shoulders reach the mat, continue to **exhale** and return your arms overhead placing your head back down to return to Step 1 position. Repeat Steps 2–7 for repetitions.

Transition: Lower your arms to your sides to prepare for the Single Leg Circles (see page 78).

modifications

If you feel any tension in your back, or you can see your abdominal muscles straining and popping out as you come up, crawl your hands up alongside your thighs to help you up.

If this still feels too difficult, do the Roll Down (see page 76) until you grow stronger and more flexible.

If you feel you are performing the Roll Up with ease, challenge yourself a little further by stretching both legs out in front of you for the whole exercise. Keep squeezing your inner thighs together throughout.

✓ **During Step 1, stay in neutral position. Be careful not to let your back arch or your ribs stick forwards as you reach overhead.**

✓ **Keep your chin towards your chest and your shoulder blades down throughout. Don't use your shoulders to come up.**

✓ **As you stretch forwards, keep the space between your hips and ribcage, so you are curved but not flopped.**

double leg stretch

body benefits

- strengthens the abominal muscles for a flatter, more toned stomach

- stretches the limbs for a more streamlined shape

- helps to improve circulation, reduce toxins in the body and promote relaxation

repetitions: 5–10

3 **Inhale**, keeping your abdominals engaged to support your spine, and stretch your body in opposite directions. Your legs extend to a 45-degree angle, while your arms lift straight behind you until they are in line with your ears. *Imagine your torso is glued to the mat as your limbs stretch away.*

2 **Exhale**, drawing in your abdominals, and roll your head and shoulders off the mat, sliding your shoulder blades down your back, your chin towards your chest. Feel your lower back lengthening along the mat.

1 Lie on your back and bend your knees in towards your chest. Your hands rest on your shins, elbows wide. **Inhale**.

precision points

✘

✘ **Don't lower your head and shoulders as you reach the arms back. Keep your chin towards your chest.**

✘ **Don't arch your back.**

caution

● Proceed with caution if you have any back or disc injuries.

● Reduce the size of the arm circles if you have a delicate shoulder.

● If you feel tension in your neck, rest your head on your head rest for a few moments, or rest your head on a couple of pillows and perform the exercise in this position until you grow stronger.

4 **Exhale**, drawing in your abdominals again as you circle your arms out to the sides, then continue the circle to bring your hands back to your shins.

5 The legs bend back in at the same time so that you return to the starting position with your head and shoulders lifted and your hands resting on your shins (Step 2). Repeat steps 3–5 for required repetitions.

Transition: Lower your head and shoulders and bend your legs so that your shins are parallel to the mat to prepare for the Single Leg Stretch (see page 86).

modifications

If you find you are arching your back, or you feel you are working into your lower back, lift your straight legs to a 90-degree angle so your toes point towards the ceiling to begin with. Gradually advance to a 45-degree angle as you get stronger.

✓ Hold your straight legs strongly together by squeezing your inner thighs.

✓ Make sure your lower back remains on the mat throughout by using your abdominal muscles.

✓ Remain still in your torso. Only your arms and legs move.

beginner's criss-cross

body benefits

- works the abdominal muscles

- trims the waist

- stretches the legs

repetitions: 5–10, alternating sides

2 **Exhale**, drawing in the abdominals as you twist from your lower ribcage to bring one elbow over to the opposite knee. As you do so, straighten your other leg out to an angle of 45 degrees.

1 Lie on your back and bend both knees in so that your thighs are at a 90-degree angle to the mat and your shins parallel to the mat. Interlace your fingers and place your hands behind your head.

Inhale, then **exhale**, drawing in the abdominals, to roll your head and shoulders off the mat, sliding the shoulder blades down the back. **Inhale** keeping the abdominals engaged.

precision points

✘ Don't twist from your shoulders but focus on twisting from your lower ribcage.

caution

● Omit this exercise if you have a back injury.

3 **Inhale**, keeping the abdominals engaged, as you twist from the lower ribcage to bring your torso back to centre, bending your straight leg in again. Make sure your elbows stay wide throughout.

4 **Exhale** as you repeat but this time twist your torso to the opposite side, straightening the other leg. *Each time imagine your torso is staked to the ground so you don't rock from hip to hip.*

Transition: Bend both knees in towards your chest and lower your head and shoulders. Lower your feet to the mat with your knees bent at a 90-degree angle. Take your arms overhead and perform a Roll-Up (see page 108) to bring yourself up to sitting in preparation for the Spine Stretch (see page 88).

modifications

If this exercise feels difficult, lower your head back to the mat on each inhalation (Step 3) until your oblique muscles grow stronger.

✓**Keep your straight leg at 45 degrees. Don't let it sink towards the floor.**

✓**Keep your elbows wide so that they don't fold inwards or touch the mat throughout.**

✓**Control the movement slowly and smoothly, don't just fling your upper body from side to side.**

corkscrew

body benefits

- strengthens the abdominals

- firms the inner thighs

- strengthens outer thighs and buttocks

- stretches the back

- improves balance

repetitions: 5 circles each side, alternating direction

1 Lie on your back with your arms by your sides. Press your palms into the mat for extra stability. Lift and straighten your legs up to the ceiling at a 90-degree angle to the mat. Turn your legs out (see page 27) engaging your lower buttock muscles throughout. Your inner thighs will also engage.

2 **Inhale** and take your legs over to one side without allowing your body to lift. *Imagine your torso is rooted to the ground.*

3 **Exhale**, drawing in the abdominals, as you circle your legs down through the centre line of your body.

precision points

✗ Don't lift your hips and keep your lower back down on the mat throughout.

✗ Don't lift your shoulders or chin.

5 Continue exhaling as you circle the knees back up and in to the centre. This movement is dynamic with the emphasis on the exhalation.

caution

● If you have a back injury, omit this exercise.

● If you feel any tension in your lower back, leave this exercise out until you grow stronger.

6 To reverse the movement: **Inhale** and take your legs over to the other side. **Exhale**, drawing in the abdominals, and circle your legs down, around and back to the centre.

Transition: Bend your legs in, then straighten them along the mat. Roll over to one side to prepare for the Double Leg Lift (see page 54).

4 Continue exhaling as you continue the circle over to the other side.

modifications

If your abdominal muscles pop out, or your back arches as you reach the low point of the circle, take your legs higher, until you are able to maintain your core stability.

As your technique improves, you can challenge yourself a little more by increasing the size of the circle without sacrificing stability.

✓Relax your neck and slide your shoulder blades down into your back to keep you stable as you circle your legs.

✓Think of reaching your legs up to the ceiling as you circle.

✓Circle your legs dynamically, with the focus on the upswing of the circle.

✓As you reach the lowest point in the circle, make sure your abdominals don't pop out, and your back doesn't arch.

side kick

body benefits

- tones the buttocks

- strengthens the hips

- trims the thighs

- streamlines your legs

repetitions: 10 each side

2 **Inhale** as you kick your top leg forwards as far as you can without shifting your torso position. In this forwards position, give a little extra beat at the top of the movement.

1 Lie on your side with one hip carefully stacked on top of the other. Your ear, the middle of your shoulder and your hip and ankle should all be in a straight line. Your feet are pointing down. Now take your legs very slightly forwards. Prop your head up on your hand making sure your elbow is in line with the rest of your body. Bend your upper arm and place your hand directly in front of you on the mat to help you balance. Make sure your shoulders are down and your neck is relaxed. Turn your legs out (see page 27) without moving your hips, engaging your lower buttock muscles. Lift your top leg a little so it is in line with your top hip.

precision points

✗ Don't allow your hips and shoulders to collapse forwards.

✗ Don't allow your leg to lift above hipbone height.

caution

● Proceed only under supervision if you have a neck or back injury.

3 **Exhale**, drawing in the abdominals, keeping your legs turned out as you swing your top leg behind you, stretching the front of the hip. *Imagine your leg swinging like a pendulum.* Make sure

you don't lean forwards as you swing, and that your leg stays in line with your hip. Just swing your leg back as far as you can without compromising your torso position.

Transition: Bend your lower leg forward for the Outer Thigh Lift (see page 56).

modifications

If you are rocking unsteadily so that you can't keep one shoulder on top of the other shoulder, and one hip on top of the

other hip, reduce the size of the kick, until you become more stable.

If you feel any pain or tension in your neck

or shoulders, or if you have delicate wrists or elbows, straighten your lower arm out along the mat and rest your head on top of it. You

can even add a cushion between your head and upper arm for additional support.

✓ **Keep the rest of your body completely still while you swing your leg back and forth, using your abdominals to keep your body stable.**

✓ **Be careful not to let your shoulders or hips move even a fraction forwards or back.**

✓ **Keep your neck long and don't sink into your shoulders.**

✓ **Think of using your buttock muscles and the muscles in the back of your thigh to swing the leg back.**

single leg kick

body benefits

● tones the back of the thighs

● stretches the often bulky front of thighs

● strengthens the back muscles

● stretches the front of the hips

● tones the arm and chest muscles

● increases spinal flexibility

repetitions: 6–10 each side, alternating sides

1 Lie on your front with your arms bent at right angles, palms flat on the mat. Your elbows should be positioned so that they lie under your shoulders, and your forearms should be parallel to each other and pressing into the mat. Lift your sternum and slide your shoulder blades down into your back. **Inhale**, then **exhale**, drawing in the abdominals, and keep your abdominals lifted throughout to protect your lower back. Squeeze your inner thighs together. **Inhale**.

precision points

✗ Don't collapse your upper torso but keep your abdominals engaged throughout.

✗ Don't lift your shoulders.

1 2 3

caution

● Omit this exercise if you have any kind of back injury or condition such as spondilolithesis.

● If you experience knee or elbow pain, omit this exercise.

● If your lower back hurts, stop immediately.

2 **Exhale**, drawing in the abdominals, and kick one leg towards your bottom, giving the leg a small extra beat at the top of the movement (near the buttocks). *Imagine you are trying to kick your buttock with your heel.*

modifications

If the kicking motion brings on cramp in your hamstrings, reduce the range of movement and move more slowly.

3 Switch and kick the other leg towards your bottom, **exhaling** at the same time. Straighten the opposite leg when it is not kicking. The inhalation between the kicks is very small, almost a sniff.

Transition: Lower your head and shoulders. Turn your head to one side and take your arms behind your back to prepare for the Double Leg Kick (see page 122).

✓Pressing your forearms into the mat and sliding your shoulder blades down your back will help keep you lifted.

✓The exercise is most beneficial at a dynamic pace. To intensify, try not to place your leg down on the mat as your leg straightens, allow it to just hover above the mat.

✓Feel your hamstrings working and your quadriceps stretching as you bend your leg, keeping your inner thighs and knees close together throughout.

✓Lengthen through the back of your neck and focus your eyes straight ahead.

double leg kick

body benefits

- strengthens the back

- opens the chest

- increases spinal flexibility

- strengthens the back of the thighs and the buttocks

- stretches the often bulky front of thighs

repetitions: 5 each side, alternating sides

2 **Exhale**, drawing the abdominals in more deeply, as you squeeze your buttocks and inner thighs together. Kick your heels towards your buttocks three times. *Imagine you are a dolphin flicking your tail to swim.*

1 Lie on your front in a straight line, resting one cheek against the mat. Interlace your fingers and clasp them behind your back taking them as close to

your shoulder blades as is comfortable while still keeping your elbows and the fronts of your shoulders down on the mat. The palms face up to the ceiling.

Inhale, then **exhale**, drawing in the abdominals and then keep them lifted throughout the exercise. **Inhale**.

precision points

✗ **Don't lift your elbows and hips off the mat.**

✓ **Remember not to release your abominals when your lift your upper body, so that your spine is protected. You should not feel any tension in the lower back.**

3

caution

● Omit this exercise if you have any kind of back injury or condition such as spondilolithesis.

● Omit this exercise if you have problem shoulders or collarbones.

● Proceed with caution if you have delicate wrists, elbows, or knees.

● Stop if you feel any pain or tension in the lower back.

3 **Inhale**, keeping the abdominals engaged, and lift your upper body off the mat, and then straighten your arms and legs.

Focus your gaze straight ahead. Your hands reach away from you so that you can feel a stretch in your pectorals.

4 **Exhale** as you lower your body, bending your arms in again and turning your cheek. **Keep exhaling** as you

bring your knees up again for the three little kicks. Repeat Steps 3–4 for required repetitions.

Transition: Roll up to a kneeling position then sit at the front of your mat for the Seal (see page 98).

modifications

If you are unable to keep your elbows and shoulders touching the mat when lying flat, lower your clasped hands to the small of your back.

5 Sit back on your heels in the Rest Position for 30 seconds (see page 63) to give your lower back a gentle stretch.

✓ **Think more of smoothly lengthening your upper body away from your hips as you lift, rather than arching your back.**

✓ **Keep the back of your neck lengthened as much as possible so that you don't crunch the back of your neck.**

✓ **Focus on using the back of your thighs and your buttock muscles to make the three little kicks.**

✓ **Make sure your legs and feet stay touching the mat while you are stretching your hands away from you past your buttocks.**

continuing the journey

You made it. You've just experienced your first thirty Pilates sessions and are now fully aware of the power of this exercise method. You look better, you feel better and you're undoubtedly hooked. Where do you go now to take it to the next level?

First of all, keep using this book. Keep practising until you can perform all the exercises fluidly. Continue to focus on the six principles and on improving your technique. By the time you've mastered the exercises in this book, you are well into Intermediate Level.

finding an instructor

If you haven't already done so, it's a good idea to book a few private classes so that a qualified Pilates instructor can check on your technique and pinpoint any imbalances you may not yet be aware of, and give you guidance as to how to improve on these.

If you want your body to improve further, you'll then need to move on to the rest of Joseph Pilates' Intermediate Level mat exercises and then on to the Advanced Level mat exercises. It would be great to enrol in a Pilates mat-class and get some supervised instruction from a qualified instructor. Mat-classes are widely available. Before you select a mat-class, you need to check out a few things first. Find out how long your instructor trained for. Most good mat training courses take about a year. Don't train with anyone who did a short course over a couple of weekends. Also, check out the size of the class. You really want a class of no more than twelve students. If the classes are too big, you won't get the supervision you are paying for.

the pilates studio

You may also want to try taking classes at a Pilates Equipment Studio. Don't panic when you first enter one. Yes, it may look as though you've walked into a medieval torture chamber but rest assured that nothing painful goes on in there. In fact, it's hugely enjoyable and deeply relaxing.

In a Pilates Studio, the Pilates mat exercises are adapted so that they can also be performed on special machines that challenge your body to a different level. These pieces of equipment were originally designed by Joseph Pilates himself and possess intriguing names like 'The Cadillac', 'The Reformer' and 'The Wunda Chair'.

When you do your routine at home on the mat, you are using gravity and your own body to provide resistance. The Pilates equipment has ropes and pulleys and springs to provide even greater resistance, allowing your body to work harder, while improving alignment. Studio classes can be taken privately or semi-privately. Semi-private classes involve taking classes in small groups in which the instructor supervises each client while the client performs his or her own personalized routine.

Far more important than the various pieces of equipment in a Pilates studio, are the instructors themselves. Under the watchful eye of a good instructor, you will be guided through a programme individually tailored to suit your strengths and weaknesses. Choose your instructor with care. As well as ensuring that they are properly qualified, you want to choose someone with whom you feel comfortable and able to ask questions of. Pilates is pretty hands-on and you want to be in a studio with an instructor who makes you feel relaxed, while challenging you to fulfill your body's potential.

Pilates will provide you with a lifetime of new challenges. You'll get the best body you can, improve your health, reduce stress, feel younger and happier. The best bit about it is you can keep doing Pilates for the rest of your days. Pilates is a personal journey. Make it yours for life!

glossary

alignment
The position of the body in which the joints of the body are in line and symmetrical.

core strength
See *core stability*.

core stability
Also referred to as girdle of strength, core strength or powerhouse, this is the band of muscles encircling the torso and extending from the lower ribcage to the pelvic floor which need to be strong to provide stability or support for the spine.

draw in the abdominals
The drawing in of the abdominal muscles, in particular the transversus abdominis, and including the pelvic floor, to effect a hollowing in the waistline.

dynamic
The movement of one part of the body as a result of the amount of energy with which you perform it.

girdle of strength
See *core stability*.

leg turn out
The engaging of the buttock muscles to effect the external rotating of the entire leg in the hip joint. If you do this correctly, the inner thigh muscles will also engage.

lengthening
A visualization to induce stretching or straightening of a muscle without tension or strain.

metabolism
The rate at which your body burns calories. Your body will burn calories even when you are not moving. You can alter your rate of metabolism by increasing your lean muscle mass and by reducing body fat.

momentum
The force with which you exert movement. Your body should not be thrown around but moved with control.

neutral spine
Position in which the natural curves of the spine are present, and in which the pubic bone and two most prominent bones at the front of the pelvis (anterior superior iliac spine) are all on one level.

opposition
The act of using a muscle or muscle group in an opposing way to another muscle or muscle group.

Pilates box
Area defined from shoulder to shoulder, shoulders to hips, and hip to hip, to act as a reference for good alignment.

powerhouse
See *core stability*.

range of motion
The scope of movement within which a muscle can be safely exercised.

scoliosis
A curvature of the spine with a lateral curve one way, and a rotation the other.

shoulder stabilization
The act of sliding or gently pressing the shoulder blades down the back, away from the ears, in order to put them into the best position for good shoulder and arm movement.

spinal articulation
The movement of the spine so that each vertebra moves individually and sequentially as you move through the spinal column.

synovial fluid
The body's version of lubrication for your joints. When you move, you increase synovial fluid production in your spine, hips, shoulders etc. to keep them flexible.

visualization
The act of holding an image in your mind to help you recruit the correct muscles for an exercise, or to help you perform it more fluidly.

index